Keto diet 30 day meal plan.
1500 calories a day

Combine with a 4 week training schedule for maximum results!

Remember that this is a meal suggestion plan. If you have an illness or disease contact your doctor or dietist.

Thank you for supporting us at dietsandworkouts.com!

In recent years, the ketogenic diet, commonly known as the keto diet, has gained significant popularity as a powerful dietary approach that offers various potential benefits for health and well-being. Characterized by its emphasis on high-fat, low-carbohydrate intake, the keto diet induces a state of ketosis in the body, where it primarily relies on fats for fuel instead of carbohydrates. While it might sound counterintuitive to traditional dietary guidelines, an increasing body of research suggests that the keto diet offers numerous advantages that extend beyond mere weight loss. In this comprehensive exploration, we delve into the science behind the ketogenic diet and its potential to promote weight management, enhance cognitive function, stabilize blood sugar levels, and improve overall metabolic health.

Keto and Weight Management

One of the most renowned benefits of the ketogenic diet is its effectiveness in aiding weight management. By drastically reducing carbohydrate intake and increasing fat consumption, the keto diet triggers a shift in the body's metabolism. As carbohydrates are limited, the body enters a state where it must rely on stored fats for energy production, leading to accelerated fat burning and, consequently, weight loss. Several studies have shown that individuals following a keto diet experience greater reductions in body weight and body mass index compared to those on traditional low-fat diets. Furthermore, the satiating nature of dietary fats helps curb appetite and reduce overall calorie consumption, contributing to sustained weight loss over time.

Cognitive Enhancement

Beyond its impact on weight, the ketogenic diet has attracted attention for its potential cognitive benefits. The brain requires a stable energy source to function optimally, and while glucose from carbohydrates is the brain's primary fuel, ketones derived from fats can also serve as an efficient energy source. The keto diet's ability to induce a state of ketosis has been linked to improved cognitive function, including enhanced focus, mental clarity, and cognitive performance. Ketones have been shown to provide a more consistent and stable energy supply to the brain, potentially reducing fluctuations in energy levels that can lead to brain fog and fatigue.

Neurological Conditions and Epilepsy

The therapeutic applications of the ketogenic diet extend beyond cognitive function. Originally developed as a medical intervention for epilepsy, the keto diet has proven highly effective in reducing the frequency and severity of seizures, particularly in drug-resistant epilepsy cases. The exact mechanisms behind its effectiveness in epilepsy treatment are still under investigation, but it is believed that the ketones' impact on neural excitability and neurotransmitter balance plays a crucial role. The success of the ketogenic diet in managing epilepsy has led to its inclusion as a recommended treatment option for epilepsy patients, showcasing its potential to address neurological conditions.

Blood Sugar Regulation and Metabolic Health

Another area where the ketogenic diet shines is in stabilizing blood sugar levels and improving metabolic health. Carbohydrates are the primary drivers of blood sugar spikes, and consistently elevated blood sugar levels can contribute to insulin resistance, a precursor to type 2 diabetes. By minimizing carbohydrate intake, the keto diet helps prevent rapid blood sugar fluctuations, reducing the demand on the body to produce excessive amounts of insulin. This can lead to improved insulin sensitivity and better blood sugar control, making the diet an attractive option for individuals with type 2 diabetes or those looking to reduce their risk of developing the condition.

Cardiovascular Health

Contrary to initial concerns about the high intake of dietary fats, research suggests that the ketogenic diet can have positive effects on cardiovascular health markers. Studies have shown that the diet can lead to significant reductions in triglyceride levels, increased levels of high-density lipoprotein (HDL) cholesterol (often referred to as "good" cholesterol), and improvements in other risk factors such as blood pressure. These findings challenge the conventional notion that dietary fat directly leads to cardiovascular issues and emphasize the importance of considering the overall dietary context.

Inflammation and Other Potential Benefits

Chronic inflammation is a common denominator in various health conditions, including autoimmune diseases, neurodegenerative disorders, and certain types of cancer. Emerging evidence suggests that the ketogenic diet may help reduce inflammation by modulating the body's inflammatory response. The diet's potential to shift the body from relying on glucose to utilizing ketones as a fuel source is believed to contribute to this anti-inflammatory effect.

Furthermore, ongoing research explores the ketogenic diet's potential applications in other areas such as cancer therapy, polycystic ovary syndrome (PCOS) management, and even longevity. While these areas are still being studied, the initial findings are promising and warrant further investigation.

Conclusion

The ketogenic diet's surge in popularity is not merely a dietary trend; it is rooted in a growing body of scientific research that supports its potential health benefits. From aiding weight management and enhancing cognitive function to stabilizing blood sugar levels and improving metabolic health, the keto diet has demonstrated multifaceted advantages that extend far beyond its initial reputation as a weight loss tool. While it might not be suitable for everyone and should be approached with careful consideration, the ketogenic diet holds promise as a viable dietary strategy for those seeking to optimize their health and well-being. As with any major dietary change, consulting with a healthcare professional is crucial to determine its appropriateness for individual needs and goals.

Shopping list for Day 1-5

- Eggs (14)
- Cheese (200g)
- Spinach (500g)
- Mushrooms (200g)
- Almonds (1 cup)
- Chicken breast (600g)
- Assorted vegetables for roasting (e.g., bell peppers, zucchini, broccoli) (800g)
- Cottage cheese (1 cup)

- Salmon fillet (400g)
- Asparagus (400g)
- Avocado (3)
- Bacon (8 slices)
- Blueberries (1 cup)
- Canned tuna (300g)
- Lettuce (1 head)
- Olive oil (4 tablespoons)
- Macadamia nuts (1 cup)
- Beef stir-fry strips (600g)
- Broccoli (400g)
- Cauliflower rice (500g)
- Almond flour (1 cup)
- Sugar-free syrup (1 bottle)
- Raspberries (1 cup)
- Grilled chicken breast (600g)
- Romaine lettuce (1 head)
- Caesar dressing (sugar-free) (4 tablespoons)
- Pork chops (600g)
- Brussels sprouts (400g)
- Greek yogurt (2 cups)
- Walnuts (1/2 cup)
- Cinnamon (1 teaspoon)
- Sunflower seeds (1/2 cup)

- Zucchini (500g)

- Pesto sauce (sugar-free) (4 tablespoons)

- Grilled shrimp (400g)

- Edamame (1 cup)

- Green beans (400g)

- Garlic (4 cloves)

- Strawberries (1 cup)

- Mixed greens (1 bag)

- Vinaigrette dressing (sugar-free) (4 tablespoons)

- Pumpkin seeds (1/2 cup)

- Cod fillet (400g)

Day 1:

- **Breakfast:** 3 egg omelette with cheese, spinach, and mushrooms (300 calories)
- **Snack:** 1/4 cup of almonds (100 calories)
- **Lunch:** Grilled chicken breast with roasted vegetables (400 calories)
- **Snack:** 1/2 cup of cottage cheese (80 calories)
- **Dinner:** Baked salmon with asparagus and butter (400 calories)
- Total calories: 1280

Day 2:

- **Breakfast**: Scrambled eggs with avocado and bacon (350 calories)
- **Snack:** 1/2 cup of blueberries (40 calories)
- **Lunch:** Tuna salad with lettuce and olive oil dressing (300 calories)
- **Snack:** 1/4 cup of macadamia nuts (200 calories)
- **Dinner:** Beef stir-fry with broccoli and cauliflower rice (400 calories)
- Total calories: 1290

Day 3:

- **Breakfast:** Keto pancakes made with almond flour and topped with sugar-free syrup (350 calories)
- **Snack:** 1/2 cup of raspberries (30 calories)
- **Lunch:** Grilled chicken Caesar salad (400 calories)
- **Snack:** 1/2 avocado with salt and pepper (150 calories)
- **Dinner:** Pork chops with roasted Brussels sprouts (400 calories)
- Total calories: 1330

Day 4:

- **Breakfast:** Greek yogurt with walnuts and cinnamon (300 calories)
- **Snack:** 1/4 cup of sunflower seeds (200 calories)
- **Lunch:** Zucchini noodles with pesto and grilled shrimp (400 calories)
- **Snack:** 1/2 cup of edamame (100 calories)
- **Dinner:** Baked chicken with green beans and garlic butter (400 calories)
- Total calories: 1400

Day 5:

- **Breakfast:** Frittata with bacon, cheese, and spinach (350 calories)
- **Snack:** 1/2 cup of strawberries (25 calories)
- **Lunch:** Grilled chicken skewers with mixed greens and vinaigrette dressing (400 calories)
- **Snack:** 1/4 cup of pumpkin seeds (200 calories)
- **Dinner:** Baked cod with roasted asparagus (400 calories)
- Total calories: 1375

Here is a shopping list for days 6-10

- Coconut milk (2 cups)

- Spinach (1.5 kg)

- Protein powder (5 scoops)

- Blackberries (1.5 cups)

- Turkey breast (750g)

- Lettuce leaves

- Avocado (4)

- Tomato (2)

- Cucumbers (2)

- Ranch dressing (sugar-free) (8 tablespoons)

- Grilled steak (800g)

- Cauliflower (2 heads)

- Almond flour bread (16 slices)

- Eggs (18)

- Bacon (16 slices)

- Cherries (2 cups)

- Grilled shrimp (800g)

- Mixed greens (2 bags)

- Lemon vinaigrette dressing (sugar-free) (8 tablespoons)

- Celery sticks

- Cream cheese (2 cups)

- Butter

- Sugar-free syrup

- Macadamia nuts (2 cups)

- Grilled chicken thighs (1.2 kg)

- Broccoli (800g)

- Cheddar cheese (2 cups)

- Small avocado (2)

- Cauliflower rice (1 kg)

- Roasted Brussels sprouts (800g)

- Feta cheese (2 cups)

- Keto bagels (16)

- Smoked salmon

- Capers

- Raspberries (2 cups)

- Turkey meatballs (750g)

- Tomato sauce (sugar-free) (1 bottle)

- Sunflower seeds (2 cups)

- Baked chicken (800g)

- Ranch dressing (sugar-free) (8 tablespoons)

Day 6:

- **Breakfast:** Keto smoothie made with coconut milk, spinach, and protein powder (350 calories)

- **Snack:** 1/2 cup of blackberries (30 calories)
- **Lunch:** Turkey lettuce wraps with avocado and tomato (300 calories)
- **Snack:** 1/2 cup of sliced cucumbers with ranch dressing (70 calories)
- **Dinner:** Grilled steak with roasted cauliflower (400 calories)
- Total calories: 1150

Day 7:

- **Breakfast:** Keto breakfast sandwich made with almond flour bread, egg, and bacon (350 calories)
- **Snack:** 1/2 cup of cherries (50 calories)
- **Lunch:** Grilled shrimp salad with mixed greens and lemon vinaigrette (400 calories)
- **Snack:** 1/2 cup of celery sticks with cream cheese (100 calories)
- **Dinner:** Baked salmon with sautéed spinach (400 calories)
- Total calories: 1300

Day 8:

- **Breakfast**: Cream cheese pancakes with butter and sugar-free syrup (350 calories)
- **Snack:** 1 oz of macadamia nuts (200 calories)
- **Lunch:** Grilled chicken thighs with broccoli and cheddar cheese (400 calories)
- **Snack:** 1 small avocado with salt and pepper (150 calories)
- **Dinner:** Baked salmon with cauliflower rice and roasted Brussels sprouts (400 calories)
- Total calories: 1500

Day 9:

- **Breakfast:** Crustless spinach and feta quiche (300 calories)
- **Snack:** 1/2 cup of blackberries (30 calories)
- **Lunch:** Grilled steak with zucchini noodles and garlic butter (400 calories)
- **Snack:** 1 oz of almonds (150 calories)
- **Dinner:** Grilled shrimp skewers with mixed greens and Caesar dressing (400 calories)
- Total calories: 1280

Day 10:

- **Breakfast:** Keto bagel with smoked salmon, cream cheese, and capers (350 calories)
- **Snack:** 1/2 cup of raspberries (30 calories)
- **Lunch:** Turkey meatballs with cauliflower rice and tomato sauce (400 calories)
- **Snack:** 1 oz of sunflower seeds (160 calories)
- **Dinner:** Baked chicken with mixed greens and ranch dressing (400 calories)
- Total calories: 1340

Here is a shopping list for days 11-14

- Eggs (16)
- Bacon (12 slices)
- Avocado (6)
- Small bell pepper (2)
- Cream cheese (1/2 cup)
- Grilled pork chops (800g)
- Assorted vegetables for roasting (e.g., bell peppers, zucchini, broccoli) (1.6kg)
- Cheddar cheese (4 oz)
- Cod fillet (800g)
- Spinach (1.5kg)
- Lemon (4)
- Butter (8 tablespoons)
- Almond milk (4 cups)

- Peanut butter (8 tablespoons)

- Chocolate protein powder (4 scoops)

- Small cucumber (2)

- Hummus (1/2 cup)

- Chicken breast (800g)

- Mixed greens (2 bags)

- Pecans (4 oz)

- Beef stir-fry strips (1.2kg)

- Broccoli (800g)

- Cauliflower rice (1kg)

- Keto waffle mix

- Sugar-free syrup

- Strawberries (1 cup)

- Canned tuna (600g)

- Olive oil (8 tablespoons)

- Walnuts (4 oz)

- Cloud bread

- Cheese (4 oz)

- Ham slices (8)

- Blueberries (1 cup)

- Grilled shrimp skewers (800g)

- Vinaigrette dressing (sugar-free) (8 tablespoons)

- Pumpkin seeds (4 oz)

Day 11:

- **Breakfast:** Scrambled eggs with bacon and avocado (350 calories)
- **Snack:** 1 small bell pepper with cream cheese (80 calories)
- **Lunch:** Grilled pork chops with roasted vegetables (400 calories)
- **Snack:** 1 oz of cheddar cheese (110 calories)
- **Dinner:** Baked cod with sautéed spinach and lemon butter (400 calories)
- Total calories: 1340

Day 12:

- **Breakfast:** Keto smoothie with almond milk, peanut butter, and chocolate protein powder (350 calories)
- **Snack:** 1 small cucumber with hummus (80 calories)
- **Lunch:** Chicken salad with mixed greens and avocado (400 calories)
- **Snack:** 1 oz of pecans (200 calories)
- **Dinner:** Beef stir-fry with broccoli and cauliflower rice (400 calories)
- Total calories: 1430

Day 13:

- **Breakfast:** Keto waffles with butter and sugar-free syrup (350 calories)
- **Snack:** 1/2 cup of strawberries (25 calories)
- **Lunch:** Tuna salad with mixed greens and olive oil dressing (300 calories)
- **Snack:** 1 oz of walnuts (200 calories)
- **Dinner:** Baked chicken with roasted asparagus and garlic butter (400 calories)
- Total calories: 1275

Day 14:

- **Breakfast:** Keto breakfast sandwich with egg, cheese, and ham on a cloud bread (350 calories)
- **Snack:** 1/2 cup of blueberries (40 calories)
- **Lunch:** Grilled shrimp skewers with mixed greens and vinaigrette dressing (400 calories)
- **Snack:** 1 oz of pumpkin seeds (170 calories)
- **Dinner:** Baked salmon with broccoli and lemon butter (400 calories)
- Total calories: 1360

Here is a shopping list for Day 15-20

- Eggs (14)
- Cheese (200g)
- Spinach (500g)
- Mushrooms (200g)
- Almonds (1 cup)
- Chicken breast (600g)
- Assorted vegetables for roasting (e.g., bell peppers, zucchini, broccoli) (800g)
- Cottage cheese (1 cup)
- Salmon fillet (400g)
- Asparagus (400g)
- Avocado (3)
- Bacon (8 slices)
- Blueberries (1 cup)
- Canned tuna (300g)
- Lettuce (1 head)
- Olive oil (4 tablespoons)
- Macadamia nuts (1 cup)
- Beef stir-fry strips (600g)
- Broccoli (400g)

- Cauliflower rice (500g)
- Almond flour (1 cup)
- Sugar-free syrup (1 bottle)
- Raspberries (1 cup)
- Grilled chicken breast (600g)
- Romaine lettuce (1 head)
- Caesar dressing (sugar-free) (4 tablespoons)
- Pork chops (600g)
- Brussels sprouts (400g)
- Greek yogurt (2 cups)
- Walnuts (1/2 cup)
- Cinnamon (1 teaspoon)
- Sunflower seeds (1/2 cup)
- Zucchini (500g)
- Pesto sauce (sugar-free) (4 tablespoons)
- Grilled shrimp (400g)
- Edamame (1 cup)
- Green beans (400g)
- Garlic (4 cloves)
- Strawberries (1 cup)
- Mixed greens (1 bag)
- Vinaigrette dressing (sugar-free) (4 tablespoons)
- Pumpkin seeds (1/2 cup)
- Cod fillet (400g)

Day 15:

- **Breakfast:** 3 egg omelette with cheese, spinach, and mushrooms (300 calories)
- **Snack:** 1/4 cup of almonds (100 calories)
- **Lunch:** Grilled chicken breast with roasted vegetables (400 calories)
- **Snack:** 1/2 cup of cottage cheese (80 calories)
- **Dinner:** Baked salmon with asparagus and butter (400 calories)
- Total calories: 1280

Day 16:

- **Breakfast:** Scrambled eggs with avocado and bacon (350 calories)
- **Snack:** 1/2 cup of blueberries (40 calories)
- **Lunch:** Tuna salad with lettuce and olive oil dressing (300 calories)
- **Snack:** 1/4 cup of macadamia nuts (200 calories)
- **Dinner:** Beef stir-fry with broccoli and cauliflower rice (400 calories)
- Total calories: 1290

Day 17:

- **Breakfast:** Keto pancakes made with almond flour and topped with sugar-free syrup (350 calories)
- **Snack:** 1/2 cup of raspberries (30 calories)
- **Lunch:** Grilled chicken Caesar salad (400 calories)
- **Snack:** 1/2 avocado with salt and pepper (150 calories)
- **Dinner:** Pork chops with roasted Brussels sprouts (400 calories)
- Total calories: 1330

Day 18:

- **Breakfast:** Greek yogurt with walnuts and cinnamon (300 calories)
- **Snack:** 1/4 cup of sunflower seeds (200 calories)
- **Lunch:** Zucchini noodles with pesto and grilled shrimp (400 calories)
- **Snack:** 1/2 cup of edamame (100 calories)
- **Dinner:** Baked chicken with green beans and garlic butter (400 calories)
- Total calories: 1400

Day 19:

- **Breakfast:** Frittata with bacon, cheese, and spinach (350 calories)
- **Snack:** 1/2 cup of strawberries (25 calories)
- **Lunch:** Grilled chicken skewers with mixed greens and vinaigrette dressing (400 calories)
- **Snack:** 1/4 cup of pumpkin seeds (200 calories)
- **Dinner:** Baked cod with roasted asparagus (400 calories)
- Total calories: 1375

Day 20:

- **Breakfast:** Keto smoothie made with coconut milk, spinach, and protein powder (350 calories)
- **Snack:** 1/2 cup of blackberries (30 calories)
- **Lunch:** Turkey lettuce wraps with avocado and tomato (300 calories)
- **Snack:** 1/2 cup of sliced cucumbers with ranch dressing (70 calories)
- **Dinner:** Grilled steak with roasted cauliflower (400 calories)
- Total calories: 1150

Here is a shopping list for days 21-26

- Coconut milk (2 cups)
- Spinach (1.5 kg)
- Protein powder (5 scoops)
- Blackberries (1.5 cups)
- Turkey breast (750g)
- Lettuce leaves
- Avocado (4)
- Tomato (2)
- Cucumbers (2)
- Ranch dressing (sugar-free) (8 tablespoons)
- Grilled steak (800g)
- Cauliflower (2 heads)
- Almond flour bread (16 slices)
- Eggs (18)
- Bacon (16 slices)
- Cherries (2 cups)
- Grilled shrimp (800g)
- Mixed greens (2 bags)
- Lemon vinaigrette dressing (sugar-free) (8 tablespoons)
- Celery sticks
- Cream cheese (2 cups)

- Butter
- Sugar-free syrup
- Macadamia nuts (2 cups)
- Grilled chicken thighs (1.2 kg)
- Broccoli (800g)
- Cheddar cheese (2 cups)
- Small avocado (2)
- Cauliflower rice (1 kg)
- Roasted Brussels sprouts (800g)
- Feta cheese (2 cups)
- Keto bagels (16)
- Smoked salmon
- Capers
- Raspberries (2 cups)
- Turkey meatballs (750g)
- Tomato sauce (sugar-free) (1 bottle)
- Sunflower seeds (2 cups)
- Baked chicken (800g)
- Ranch dressing (sugar-free) (8 tablespoons)

Day 21:

- **Breakfast:** Keto breakfast sandwich made with almond flour bread, egg, and bacon (350 calories)
- **Snack:** 1/2 cup of cherries (50 calories)
- **Lunch:** Grilled shrimp salad with mixed greens and lemon vinaigrette (400 calories)
- **Snack:** 1/2 cup of celery sticks with cream cheese (100 calories)
- **Dinner:** Baked salmon with sautéed spinach (400 calories)
- Total calories: 1300

Day 22:

- **Breakfast:** Cream cheese pancakes with butter and sugar-free syrup (350 calories)
- **Snack:** 1 oz of macadamia nuts (200 calories)
- **Lunch:** Grilled chicken thighs with broccoli and cheddar cheese (400 calories)
- **Snack:** 1 small avocado with salt and pepper (150 calories)
- **Dinner:** Baked salmon with cauliflower rice and roasted Brussels sprouts (400 calories)
- Total calories: 1500

Day 23:

- **Breakfast:** Crustless spinach and feta quiche (300 calories)
- **Snack:** 1/2 cup of blackberries (30 calories)
- **Lunch:** Grilled steak with zucchini noodles and garlic butter (400 calories)
- **Snack:** 1 oz of almonds (150 calories)
- **Dinner:** Grilled shrimp skewers with mixed greens and Caesar dressing (400 calories)
- Total calories: 1280

Day 24:

- **Breakfast:** Keto bagel with smoked salmon, cream cheese, and capers (350 calories)
- **Snack:** 1/2 cup of raspberries (30 calories)
- **Lunch:** Turkey meatballs with cauliflower rice and tomato sauce (400 calories)
- **Snack:** 1 oz of sunflower seeds (160 calories)
- **Dinner:** Baked chicken with mixed greens and ranch dressing (400 calories)
- Total calories: 1340

Day 25:

- **Breakfast:** Scrambled eggs with bacon and avocado (350 calories)
- **Snack:** 1 small bell pepper with cream cheese (80 calories)
- **Lunch:** Grilled pork chops with roasted vegetables (400 calories)
- **Snack:** 1 oz of cheddar cheese (110 calories)
- **Dinner:** Baked cod with sautéed spinach and lemon butter (400 calories)
- Total calories: 1340

Day 26:

- **Breakfast:** Keto smoothie with almond milk, peanut butter, and chocolate protein powder (350 calories)
- **Snack:** 1 small cucumber with hummus (80 calories)
- **Lunch:** Chicken salad with mixed greens and avocado (400 calories)
- **Snack:** 1 oz of pecans (200 calories)
- **Dinner:** Beef stir-fry with broccoli and cauliflower rice (400 calories)
- Total calories: 1430

Here is a shopping list for days 27-30

- Eggs (16)
- Bacon (12 slices)
- Avocado (6)
- Small bell pepper (2)
- Cream cheese (1/2 cup)
- Grilled pork chops (800g)
- Assorted vegetables for roasting (e.g., bell peppers, zucchini, broccoli) (1.6kg)
- Cheddar cheese (4 oz)
- Cod fillet (800g)
- Spinach (1.5kg)
- Lemon (4)
- Butter (8 tablespoons)
- Almond milk (4 cups)
- Peanut butter (8 tablespoons)
- Chocolate protein powder (4 scoops)
- Small cucumber (2)
- Hummus (1/2 cup)
- Chicken breast (800g)
- Mixed greens (2 bags)
- Pecans (4 oz)
- Beef stir-fry strips (1.2kg)
- Broccoli (800g)
- Cauliflower rice (1kg)
- Keto waffle mix

- Sugar-free syrup
- Strawberries (1 cup)
- Canned tuna (600g)
- Olive oil (8 tablespoons)
- Walnuts (4 oz)
- Cloud bread
- Cheese (4 oz)
- Ham slices (8)
- Blueberries (1 cup)
- Grilled shrimp skewers (800g)
- Vinaigrette dressing (sugar-free) (8 tablespoons)
- Pumpkin seeds (4 oz)

Day 27:

- **Breakfast:** Keto waffles with butter and sugar-free syrup (350 calories)
- **Snack:** 1/2 cup of strawberries (25 calories)
- **Lunch:** Tuna salad with mixed greens and olive oil dressing (300 calories)
- **Snack:** 1 oz of walnuts (200 calories)
- **Dinner:** Baked chicken with roasted asparagus and garlic butter (400 calories)
- Total calories: 1275

Day 28:

- **Breakfast:** Keto breakfast sandwich with egg, cheese, and ham on a cloud bread (350 calories)
- **Snack:** 1/2 cup of blueberries (40 calories)
- **Lunch:** Grilled shrimp skewers with mixed greens and vinaigrette dressing (400 calories)
- **Snack:** 1 oz of pumpkin seeds (170 calories)
- **Dinner:** Baked salmon with broccoli and lemon butter (400 calories)
- Total calories: 1360

Day 29:

- **Breakfast:** Mushroom and spinach omelette with cheddar cheese (350 calories)
- **Snack:** 1 oz of pistachios (160 calories)
- **Lunch:** Keto chicken and vegetable soup (350 calories)
- **Snack:** 1 small bell pepper with cream cheese (80 calories)

- **Dinner:** Baked pork tenderloin with roasted radishes and garlic butter (400 calories)
- Total calories: 1340

Day 30:

- **Breakfast:** Keto smoothie bowl with unsweetened coconut milk, berries, and almond butter (350 calories)
- **Snack:** 1 oz of cashews (160 calories)
- **Lunch:** Grilled shrimp salad with mixed greens, avocado, and cilantro lime dressing (400 calories)
- **Snack:** 1 small cucumber with hummus (80 calories)
- **Dinner:** Baked chicken thighs with roasted cauliflower and Parmesan cheese (400 calories)
- Total calories: 1390

Thank you for supporting us at dietsandworkouts.com!
You can combine our meal plans with a 4 week workout plan for maximum effect!

Printed in Great Britain
by Amazon

27743741R00020